The Essential C

Beginners

Healthy Delicious Recipes, Meal Plans, Gain Muscle, Lose weight, Shed Fat and Maintain Hormonal Balance in Women for a Healthier Life

By

Rina S. Gritton

Acknowledgements

This book could not have been written without the guidance and generosity of many people. To all of you who encouraged and stood by me, thank you.

Copyright © 2019 Rina S. Gritton

The author retains all rights. No part of this document may be reproduced or transmitted in any form or by any means, electronic or mechanical, including photocopying, recording, or by any information storage and retrieval system without permission in writing from the author. The unauthorized reproduction or distribution of this copyrighted work is illegal.

DISCLAIMER

This guide is not a replacement for competent medical advice from qualified Healthcare personnel. It is intended to provide information to aid you with cooking healthy and delicious meals at any time of the day.

I put down this book to provide you with skills and information to enable you to attain your desired physical and mental goals through some simple recipes.

Contents

CHAPTER ONE 6

What is Carb Cycling? 6

The Transformation of Protein into Muscle 10

The Know-how 10

Consume the fiber 11

Even out the Macros 11

A count of the needed calories 12

Eat well on all days 12

Keto and Low Carb days 13

Who is Carb Cycling Meant For? 14

CHAPTER TWO 17

How Effective is Carb Cycling as a Dietary Practice? 17

Constant moderate re-feeds 19

Inconstant large intake of carbs 20

Strategic Carb Cycling 20

Carb Cycling for Muscle Growth 21

Can you Lose Weight? 22

Improving Muscle Growth 23

Carb Cycling and Weight Loss 25

Protein and Weight Loss 26

Side Effects 28

Hormonal imbalance in women 29

Carb Cycling and Hormone Balance 32

Relieving of PMS 33

Fat for Hormone Balance 34

Improving Sexual and Reproductive Health 35

Improvement in Insulin Sensitivity 35

Reduction in Cortisol Levels 36

Balancing Hormones with Carb Cycling 37

Daily intake of Protein 38

Stay away from highly processed carbs 39

Eat Healthy Fats 40

Green Tea 41

Exercise 42

Increase your intake of fatty fish 44

Avoid Carbonated Sugary Drinks 44

Take control of stress 45

Have Quality Sleep Times 46

Eat Eggs 47

Eat Reasonably 47

Fiber Diet 48

CHAPTER THREE 49

Ways of Carrying out Carb Cycling 49

Why is Carb Cycling Important? 49

How to Carb Cycle 51

Ascertain your calorie and carb needs 52

Even Day Spread 52

Formulating a meal plan 53

Keeping Records 54

Consulting your Medical Practitioner 55

The Good Carb 55

Cheat once in a while 56

Eat in the Morning 57

Identify the Challenges 57

Getting a Grip on What Carb Cycling is 58

Calorie Cycling is Carb Cycling 59

Foods to Eat and Avoid 59

Foods to eat when Carb Cycling 62

CHAPTER FOUR 63

Meal Planning 63

Eat regularly, at least five times a day 64

Whole foods 65

Fiber 65

Protein 65

Omega 3 Fatty Acids 66

The Stumbling Blocks 66

Plan your meals 67

Eat your calories 67

Make use of spices 68

CHAPTER FIVE 69

Setting up the Carb Cycling Sample Diet Plan 69

The No Carb Days 69

The Low Carb Days 70

The Moderate Carb Days 70

The High Carb Days 70

Sample High Carb Diet Plan 71

Carb Cycling Diet for Body Composition
Maintenance or Muscle Building 74

High Carb Fruits 75

High Carb Grains 76

High Carb Vegetables 76

CHAPTER SIX 85

The Ultimate Food List 85

Other Books by the Author 97

The Healing Path with Essential CBD oil and Hemp oil: The Simple Beginner's Guide to Managing Anxiety Attacks, Weight Loss, Diabetes and Holistic Healing 97

Cannabis Bud Smoothie: Healthy Medicinal Drinks and Marijuana Infusions 100

Cannabis Cultivation and Horticulture: The Simple Guide to Growing Marijuana Indoors Using Hydroponics 101

The Complete Instant Pot Cookbook: Simple Ketogenic Diet Cookbook Recipes, The Simple Slow Cooker Cookbook and The Healthy Crock Pot Cookbook 104

CHAPTER ONE

What is Carb Cycling?

The fashion of what we eat and the techniques employed in how we take in nutrition comes in circles. Folks used to avoid fats and then embraced it. The focus is now is no or little amount of carbs. As the research on how the intake of different classes of foods affects the human body, there is bound to be more changes in how we reach out to the food around us.

The terror that carbs strike into the heart of the health-conscious individual is somewhat profound. This is because when you take a closer look at the regular meals an individual eats daily, carbohydrates take a massive chunk. From the highly processed foods containing large amounts of white flour such as bread, pastries to carbonated drinks can be cause for concern if you are particular about weight, health, and where you see yourself health-wise in the next few years.

You might have considered avoiding all forms of carbs from your diet based on the bad rap this class of food is getting. That would be a wrong decision because carbohydrates also perform essential functions in the human body, and cutting it out will most likely have dire consequences. If you are in a dilemma on how to go about handling your carbohydrate intake, focus more on reducing the consumption to a more "reasonable" amount and consume more of complex carbs that have a low glycemic index e.g., brown rice, vegetables, and oats. Such forms of carbs release the energy needed for your daily activities and for workouts if you have included that in your weight loss regime. To ensure that your carb intake is not jeopardized, carb cycling comes in. This is a method of consuming high carb-containing foods on certain days and taking in of low amount of carbs on other days.

Carb cycling is an avenue through which you can eat foods that you actually love and have this mindset that you are not on a diet during certain days of the week. The crust of the diet plan is that does it have any effect on your weight gain and sustainability in the long term? We will get to that later in the book.

In carb cycling, you alternate the days during which you take in large amounts of carbs and days in which the intake of carbs is low. This is the pattern that is adopted, and it depends on how active you intend to be during each day. The concept behind carb cycling is quite firm based on the physical activity levels on each day of the week. You get to take in high carb amounts on days when you are going to be exerted with exercises and other activities, and on days when you plan to take it slow, your carb intake will be significantly reduced. Exercising makes use of the body's carbs reservoir to fuel that activity making for a perfect fit for your high carb days. This creates a massive amount of energy available for your workout session, and you can extend your physical activity for a more extended period and burning more energy reserves. This doesn't mean that you shouldn't consume any form of calories on your off days, rather, the amount should be moderate to build up the lost energy and not make you feel as if you are cutting out any major food class and the delights that come with the eating process. The amount of carbs you consume on the alternate days is not set in stone. This is primarily determined by your weight loss goal target and the type of physical activities that you have set for each day. Not minding the varying types of carb cycling diet types, your carb consumption should be a personalized design specific to your own goals.

The main idea on which carb cycling is built is that when your carb intake is reduced on certain days, the fat reservoir is dipped into as the body's source of energy. This is an essential avenue for managing your weight, increasing the fuel storage of the carbs for when it is needed, and also increasing your body fat loss. With a well-planned strategy of your high and low carb days, you can adequately increase your endurance and energy outputs on days of high physical activities.

The Transformation of Protein into Muscle

The Know-how

With carb cycling, there is the need for you to invest a bit more of your time compared to some of the other diet plans out there. You will need to continually take measurements of your body weight, calorie intake, etc. If you are an individual who is free-spirited and doesn't like to be held down with too many rules, this diet type is almost certainly not for you. On the other hand, if you don't mind following the rules that make up the building blocks of the carb cycling diet, then you will most definitely reap the benefits that come along with it. Let's take a peep at some of the vital information that makes carb cycling what it is.

Consume the fiber

On days when your carbohydrate intake is going to be reduced is not an avenue for you to avoid taking your vegetables. This day is one in which you cut out harmful over-processed, high glycemic index foods such as white sugar, polished rice, etc. Eat your vegetable, quinoa, grains, oats, and fruits, etc. that are high in fiber

Even out the Macros

For every meal that you will be taking, find a balance between the major classes of macronutrients in your diet; protein, fats, and carbs. The fat component has the highest ration, while the protein and carbs are evenly distributed. In your meals, the protein content should be at about one gram for every kilogram of your body weight. On days when your carb intakes are high, the amount of carbs would be increased while the fat and protein levels remain unchanged. However, on the low carb days, the carb intake will witness a reduction with the fat and protein contents not changing. The goal here is to create an atmosphere of you not noticing the reduced carb intake.

A count of the needed calories

It is necessary to have in mind a maximum calorific intake every day and try as much as possible to meet it. Take this method, if you aim to get rid of the excess body weight, you will have to multiply your body weight by ten, and the result is the number of calories you will consume every day. On the other hand, if you are ok with your current weight and would want it to remain the same, multiply your body weight by twelve, or if you want an increase in your body weight, multiply it by fifteen.

Eat well on all days

You need the energy from the carbs, your body system, and your brain needs the simple sugar to burn and function quickly. In the absence of glucose, which is the most accessible and most readily available source of energy, your body looks for alternative sources of energy e.g., protein. This will be a counterproductive path if you aim to bulk up and build some muscle mass. Eat carbs even on your low carb consuming days. It will also prevent you from becoming tired quickly during the day.

Keto and Low Carb days

The Keto diet is quite strict when it comes to the number of specific foods that you can eat and what you are allowed to eat. The principle here is based on high-fat consumption and a deficient intake of carbs to bring your body into ketosis through the formation of ketones. If you fail to cut down on your intake of carbs drastically, your body will simply move from the fuel source of ketones to glucose, thus taking your body out of ketosis, and the whole essence of the diet would have been lost.

In carb cycling low carb days, there is no binding rules or specific answer to how much or what you can eat. The "rules" vary with individual goals, but the baseline here is to limit your carb intake to around one hundred and fifty grams of carbs per day as compared to the keto diet which is almost less than one-third of this amount.

Who is Carb Cycling Meant For?

This dietary approach is mainly focused on two categories of people; folks who are engaged in low carb diets and those who are sportsmen or women.

If your goal is to lose some weight, carb cycling is a healthy approach. Carbs are the primary source of fuel when you are physically active or exercising and when you increase your intake of carbs just before your exercise regime, and after a hard work out session, you will derive the best from the dietary approach. If your workout session is a high-intensity program, the likelihood is that the energy released during the process will be significantly reduced on a low carb diet; in this case, a carb cycling process can come to your aid by increasing the number of carbs needed to complete the exercise.

For individuals who are active in sports or professional athletes, reducing the intake of carbs just before the onset of major competitions is beneficial towards the storage of glycogen for the time when the high levels of carbs are then consumed. The reduction of carbs when in training helps the body adjust correctly for when the high level of carbs are consumed when a high level of performance is most needed.

Some elements of carb cycling can be found integrated into the keto diet, but you don't necessarily have to consume relatively high amounts of fats to reap all the amazing benefits that this diet has. The carb cycling can be fitted right into any type of diet you are on.

If you are on a keto diet, it is not advisable that you cycle your carbs. The lowering and increasing of your carb intake will move your body out of ketosis. If, however, you would still love to cycle your crabs while on the keto diet, try to limit the high carb days to at most two times in a week. The aim of the keto diet is to use fat storage in your body as the main source of fuel through ketosis. When you then continuously move in and out of ketosis, the goal of the process would have been negated, and it can be tough trying to actually know if the diet is perfectly fitted for your body.

If the principles of the diet plan are maintained, it can be used by everyone for a regulated period. Due to the "tough" rules of the program that must be stuck with, and it is most likely that individuals who have nutritional problems are not best fitted to practice carb cycling. Carb cycling is the last resort and should only be engaged when other dietary approaches have been exhausted.

CHAPTER TWO

How Effective is Carb Cycling as a Dietary Practice?

Altering the carb intake towards bulking up, weight loss, improved endurance is on the increase and won't be going away anytime soon. Your weight goals, nutritional balance, and fitness are mostly centered on eating the correct amount and type of carbs at any given time. A few examples of diets out there have gone a step further by cutting out carbohydrates as a way of preventing the accumulation of fats and losing weight. This, however, is unhealthy and may have dire consequences. The nature of carbohydrates has been confounding both dieticians and the general public due to the fashion diets and restrictions surrounding it. For any dietary method, you have decided to employ in staying fit, bulking up on lean muscle and improving your endurance levels, there is the need to look at the inclusion of carbs holistically in the whole process. You should, however, note that the amount of carbohydrate to be incorporated into the meal of any one individual is different from person to person.

You might just be getting to know about carb cycling after your extensive research on healthy ways to lose weight, but I can categorically tell you that this diet type has been around for a long while now.

For proper cycling of carbs in your daily meals, there is a need for you to have an idea of the rough estimate of carbs that you should be consuming. There are several factors that will determine the number of carbs to be involved in the cycling process.

The level of your physical activity

Your age

Height

Weight

Your Basal metabolic rate

Your intake of essential macros

Carb cycling ideally should not be used for an extended period. The weight control plan that you have planned for your body should not be focused totally on carb cycling. It should be used only after you have tried other diet practices, and that doesn't work for you.

The major approaches of this diet type are;

Constant moderate re-feeds

In this method, a day is inserted into the regular three to four days of the reduced carb intake period. On this day that you have picked, your carb intake would be significantly higher compared to the other days of low carb intake. This technique works best for folks who have a hard time cutting carbs from their diets for a long time.

Inconstant large intake of carbs

A day is picked after a period of low carb intake, which can range from a week to two weeks for you to consume a large number of carbs. This large intake of carbs after a long time of abstinence is compensation for your steadfastness to the diet plan. This brings your body to the brink of starvation, close enough but not pushed over the edge into full-blown starvation.

Strategic Carb Cycling

Here, you have a well-regulated menu list, which consists of moderate carb consumption at fixed periods on days of low carb consumption. This method is a deviation from a high intake of high carb due to the fluid nature of the menu. It gives room for your metabolic system to be always a step behind and sometimes matches your nutritional intake.

Carb Cycling for Muscle Growth

For muscle gains, there is a need to exceed the amount of calorie burnt each day, i.e., a surplus of calories is needed. This is a dicey situation because if this condition is maintained for an extended time, there is the probability that there will be an accumulation of fat. To negate this potential downside, carb cycling comes in. The menu is formulated in such a way to partner with the daily physical activities to set up an environment of abundant calories in the system.

On days in which your intake of carbs is significantly increased, you must make it a point of note to exercise to fully reap the benefits of the surge of fuel in your system.

The low carb days improves the body's sensitivity to insulin, encourages progressive weight loss, and obviously burns fats. On the other side of the coin, days of large carb intakes provide a surge of fuel needed for muscular activities and also including the moderating of hormones responsible for your appetite; grehlin and leptin.

If your diet plan is appropriately structured and kept for a relatively brief period, the positive health effects on the body can be immeasurable. You should be disciplined enough to eat foods that contain whole nutrients while at the same time, avoid overly processed food items.

Your body undergoes a deficit in calories, which is a pathway through which weight loss occurs. You should, however, pay attention to how much carbs you take in, in relation to your weight at all times. This will act as a barrier from allowing your body to become comfortable and embracing this form of nutrition availability fully.

Can you Lose Weight?

The correlation between the insulin levels in your blood and carbohydrate consumption is a fact that has been researched and confirmed to be true.

With a consistently high level of insulin in the blood, the probability of body weight increase is also high. This is a major stumbling block to your weight loss progress.

A healthy cut back on the carb intake and a deficit in the caloric values of your meals brings about an improvement in the sensitivity of insulin in the body. Alternating the carb intake is a perfect way of staying healthy overall.

Improving Muscle Growth

Carb cycling is the in thing with sportsmen and has been used to build a store of energy through the accumulation of carbs to encourage muscle growth. In training, athletes focus on reducing and increasing the number of carbs that they consume.

A healthy alteration of the intake of carbs brings about a muscle build-up against unwanted fat accumulation. If you are interested in muscle gain and fat burn out, this diet demands an almost absolute focus in setting up your daily food intake is needed from you in monitoring the amount of energy you will be consuming during the course of the coming days. Carbs are not the only major focus of the diet plan during this phase; other food categories are also looked into in details e.g., the number of fats and protein that are present in your meal at each time.

For muscle growth, it is quite evident that you have to consume a more substantial proportion of protein when making use of the carb cycling diet practice. Its percentage content of every meal should range between thirty-five to forty percentage based on your end muscle goals. On the other hand, your carb intake should not exceed fifteen percent of your meal at any one time.

Health Advantages

Muscle recovery

Insulin regulation

Mental wellbeing

Improves the metabolic rate

Promotes weight loss

Increased energy availability

Regulation of hormones

The advantages of carb cycling also extend to persons dealing with type 2 diabetes, insulin-resistance, battling with weight loss, and prediabetics.

Carb Cycling and Weight Loss

The major reason why a lot of people embrace carb cycling is to reduce their ever-increasing body weight. The question here is, does carb cycling have any positive impact on the weight of an individual? Yes, it does because as with any dietary practice that involves the restriction of calories for a predetermined period setting up a deficit in the calorie intake, weight loss is bound to occur notwithstanding the type of foods you eat and how you have designed your eating pattern. The endpoint simply means that a constant intake of fewer calories than what your body makes use of will result in a weight loss. With this in mind, the carb cycling diet plan is not another fad, it is the path to toe if you aim to lose weight the healthy way.

Protein and Weight Loss

The relatively higher intake of protein against a commensurate reduction in crab consumption brings about a "Thermic Effect of Food" (TEF). The TEF is the needed energy by the body to take in food substances, break it down, absorb, and also store it. This process requires about one-tenth of the daily energy consumption for a typical body type, and it is termed the "Total Daily Energy Expenditure" (TDEE). There is a difference between the TEF and TDEE because of the type of macros in your meal due to the fact that the macros (fat, protein, and carbohydrates) all have TEF values that differ from one another. The protein component of your food needs a much higher TEF value to break it down and store (about thirty-five percent), fat (less than three percent), and carbs (fifteen percent). This point to the fact why diets containing a high amount of protein are desirable in the burning of fat and weight loss and why when you consume a high-fat diet against a diet high in carbs, you will gain weight a bit faster.

If a more significant percentage of the food you eat every day is in the form of proteins, your body will burn a lot of energy in the form of TEF to breakdown and store the protein. This will keep your body in a calorific deficit.

The intake of a relatively low amount of protein during your weight loss program can also bring about a loss of muscle mass. This defeats the burning of fat through the following;

A cut back on the number of calories expended during physical activities

A disruption of the metabolic process

Reduction in the basal metabolic rate

To avoid the above, it is best to consume a healthy size of protein in your meals.

Side Effects

In the beginning, when you start with carb cycling and the low carb days, it is most likely that you will experience cravings for carbs, moodiness and easily irritated, constipation, sleep disturbances, etc. due to your body making use of the store of carbs that it has left. These symptoms and changes that you experience are called the carb flu, and it is only for a short while. Once you begin to consume healthy amounts of fluids and electrolytes, it will pass quickly.

The body systems of individuals are different and will react in different ways to environmental conditions and the alterations of the intake of nutrients. With carb cycling, people with pre-existing conditions such as autoimmune hypothyroidism (Hashimoto's syndrome) will see a reduction in the metabolic function and functioning of the thyroid. People with eating disorders, breastfeeding, pregnant should not under any circumstances practice carb cycling. Other side effects include and are not limited to;

Decreased testosterone

Reduced immune function

Increased cortisol production

Affected cognitive functions

Hormonal imbalance in women

The downside of restricting the intake of carbs for an extended period can bring about an upheaval in the hormonal system of anybody and women mostly. This is because of the sensitive nature of the body of a woman to the scarce macronutrient or an overabundance, which may be related to having body fat, which helps in the process of procreation of new offspring.

The body has several organs that produce hormones that are either general in their actions or specific. The Central Nervous System, however, is responsible for the control of all the hormonal systems in the body. In the brain can be found the pituitary and hypothalamus, which are extremely sensitive to the lack of or presence of energy for its functioning. These two hormonal glands do not work in isolation; they function closely with other glands in the body, such as the adrenal gland.

When a lady restricts her carbohydrate or calorie intake for a very long time or there is even if the lady consumes the right amount of calories with no sufficient carbohydrates, there is the likelihood that she will come down with hypothalamic amenorrhea. This disorder results in an irregular menstrual cycle, and the hormonal system starts to yo-yo.

The normal levels of hormones in the body drop drastically, sending shockwaves around the body. The follicle-stimulating hormone (FSH), luteinizing hormone, testosterone, estrogen, and progesterone becomes decreased in the system. An increase in the intake of carbohydrates also brings about a spike in the production of cortisol, which relates stimulus to the pituitary gland through the HPA axis to reduce its functions. The HPA axis, which comprises of the hypothalamus and the adrenal gland, is responsible for the regulation of your mood, response to stress, libido, digestion, immune system, energy levels, and metabolism.

Both ladies and guys all want to get healthy and more muscle mass by eating low carb diets for long periods. This can cause a change in the hormonal system, most notably in ladies who are still in their prime. Here are some of the potential dangers that ladies can face;

Blood sugar swings and hypoglycemia

Increased body fat

Irregular menstrual cycle

Mental health challenges

Loss of bone density

Chronic inflammation

Lethargy

Sleep deprivation

These are certainly not the goals of you going on a low carb cycling diet.

Carb Cycling and Hormone Balance

With all the advantages that this diet type has, the least talked about and also as important as the weight loss aspect is the hormonal balance duties that it performs. When the carb cycling diet is followed the healthy way diligently, the out of sync hormonal system can be restored. Low sex drive, PMS, menopause, mood swings, and other imbalances can be checked when you eat right.

Your carb cycling diet can help balance your hormones in the following ways;

Relieving of PMS

When a lady is experiencing PMS, several effects such as depression, fatigue, hot flashes can be felt, which are not so wholesome and can negatively affect the quality of life. This syndrome is due to having an abundance of estrogen in the system with a minimal level of progesterone. This situation can be caused by having a diet having a high amount of processed carbs. PMS or estrogen abundance in the body is also as a result of toxic alternates that are all around us. These forms of estrogens do not just bring about the uncomfortable side effects associated with PMS; they can also be precursors to autoimmune diseases, cancer, infertility, etc. To stay on top of the situation and to manage it appropriately, consume more wholesome vegetables with lots of spices and herbs that will help cleanse and detoxify your body.

Fat for Hormone Balance

The inclusion of a healthy amount of fat in your diet in conjunction with protein and carbs is essential for improving and maintaining a healthy hormonal system. Some sources of healthy fats to be consumed are olive oil, coconut oil, avocados, butter, nuts and seeds, oily fish, and other foods with healthy fat content. Fats are essential in the production of the biochemical substances called hormones as they serve as the starting materials for progesterone, testosterone, and estrogen.

Improving Sexual and Reproductive Health

When the sex hormones in the body of a lady are not in equilibrium, there is the possibility of the development of polycystic ovary syndrome (PCOS). When a statistic was taken of the ladies suffering from this condition, it was discovered that they have poor blood sugar control, insulin resistance, and are overweight. Tackling this syndrome is a lifelong battle that can be managed with the intake of diets rich in fats and protein.

Improvement in Insulin Sensitivity

The levels of carbs consumed on both low carb and high carb days assist in maintaining a balance in the insulin levels in the body. The hormone insulin is in charge of blood sugar levels in the body. It is not only linked to the control of blood sugar, but there is also a correlation between it and the sex hormones. With the proper diet, your body becomes insulin sensitive, and equilibrium is found and maintained. With the balance in place, you will begin to experience the upside of your diet. There will be a lowered risk of heart diseases, the hot flashes will reduce or totally fade away, reduction in the chances of Alzheimer's, loss of bone matter will be stopped with an increase in bone health, improved energy levels, and so much more.

Reduction in Cortisol Levels

The adrenal glands are designed to act as a check and balance for stresses that we face every day by secreting the hormone cortisol into the bloodstream. This hormone helps in the release of energy to help the body cope with whatever immediate challenges it might be facing. Due to the high-stress levels that modern society forces the body to go through regularly, day in, day out, there is the probability that the adrenal glands are on hyper mode, constantly releasing cortisol into the body. The abundant levels of this hormone in the body prevent the formation and action of other essential hormones such as estrogen, progesterone, and testosterone. This ultimately results in the loss of much-needed equilibrium in the levels of sex hormones, low libido, muscle mass loss, and high blood sugar.

Managing this, try to increase your intake of vegetables that are low in carbohydrates such as kale, green vegetables, cauliflower, parsley, broccoli, etc.

Balancing Hormones with Carb Cycling

Hormones are biochemical messengers that have monumental impacts on the body in varying ways, from the physical to the mental. They are active in taking charge of mood, appetite, etc. There are specific glands that secrete a precise amount of hormone into the body based on how much is needed at any one time. In this jet age, with a lot of changes in the diet and environment, the hormonal imbalance has become the order of the day. In addition to this, as we grow older, the number of hormones needed for normal body functioning also decreases, and this varies from person to person.

It is not all gloom and doom as taking control of your lifestyle and how and what you eat has an impact on your hormonal balance. To balance your hormones and be in top health all the time, I will be touching on a few ways through which you can naturally balance your hormones through carb cycling.

Daily intake of Protein

The intake of a healthy portion of protein on a regular basis in every meal is crucial. Proteins are a source of essential amino acids which are so-called because your body cannot synthesize it and need it to come from foods that you eat for proper body functioning. The duty of protein includes maintenance of the skin, muscle growth, hormonal balance, etc. Some of the hormones secreted control your urge to eat. A healthy portion of protein during your meals will substantially depress the need to eat because there is a reduction of the hormone related to hunger; ghrelin and there is the release of the hormone that gives you the feeling of being satisfied and full; GLP-1 and PYY. For optimum production of these hormones, ensure that you consume at least thirty grams of protein during any mealtime.

Stay away from highly processed carbs

Studies have shown that overly processed carbs can cause detrimental effects to the human body. You should aim to reduce the intake of foods in these categories to the barest minimum in order to boost and maintain the production of hormones and cut down the risks of severe health challenges.

Simple sugars such as glucose and fructose are found in a lot of processed foods and honey, corn syrup, and maple syrup. When it is consumed for a long time can always bring about spikes in the insulin levels, encourage insulin resistance mostly in folks with excess weight problems and diabetics. Diets that have a large proportion of white flour products will ultimately bring about insulin resistance in the persons.

On the other hand, a low or medium carb diet, which is more focused on the consumption of whole foods, will most likely reduce the incidence of insulin resistance on obese or overweight individuals. Other health variables linked to insulin levels, such as polycystic ovary syndrome, can also be managed with the intake of whole food carbs instead of overly refined sugars.

Eat Healthy Fats

When you eat foods high in healthy fats, there will be the production of hormones that will suppress hunger and also assist in the reduction of insulin resistance.

The type of fats that you should be eating on a regular basis are the medium-chain triglycerides (MCTs), which are absorbed straight away by the liver to be used as a source of fuel. Sources of medium-chain triglycerides include palm oil, coconut oil, etc. Other fat sources that help in increasing insulin sensitivity are nuts and dairy fats.

Stay away from Trans-fat as they encourage insulin resistance and the deposit of fat around the mid-region of the body.

Green Tea

If you have been on the lookout for a beverage that will boost your metabolism, I am here to let you know that green tea is a perfect fit. It is packed full of antioxidants (epigallocatechin gallate; EGCG), which has massive beneficial effects on the human body. A regular intake of green tea will lower insulin levels and bring about an increase in insulin sensitivity in individuals who are diabetic and overweight. For improved insulin response and the associated health benefits, aim to drink at least one cup of green tea a day.

Exercise

Regular and well structured physical activities have a positive, healthy impact on the health of humans. One of the significant benefits to be derived from exercising is the increased insulin sensitivity, and a cut down on insulin levels. Elevated levels of insulin in the body are detrimental, but a moderate amount at any given time serves a balancing function by aiding the cells of the body to absorb amino acids and sugars which are used as fuel.

When the insulin levels in the body becomes too high, some of the health effects that can develop includes; diabetes, inflammation, cancer, and cardiac problems. All these are linked to insulin resistance, which develops as a result of your cells not reacting as they should to the messages sent by the hormone.

When exercising becomes a part of your lifestyle, there will be improved levels of the hormone adiponectin, which controls your metabolism and fights inflammation. Hormones which also fights the effects of aging on the muscles are produced continuously in healthy amounts.

Some exercises that help in improving insulin sensitivity and cut down on the amount of insulin are endurance exercises, aerobics, and strength training. Not everyone can engage in moderate or highly physical activities. If you fall into this category, you can take up walking. Brisk walking several times a week will greatly improve your quality of life if adhered to for an extended period of time.

Increase your intake of fatty fish

Fatty fishes have high contents of omega-3 fatty acids and are quite good at tackling inflammation. For the maintenance of hormonal balance, decreasing stress levels, and a reduction of the hormones adrenaline and cortisol, a healthy intake of fatty fishes, is advised. Examples of fishes that fall in this category are sardines, mackerel, salmon, and herring.

Avoid Carbonated Sugary Drinks

Refined sugars, most especially when in the fluid form, can be devastating to the human body. They encourage insulin resistance in overweight individuals. When there is regular consumption of sugary drinks, there is the likelihood that you will take in far more calories than your body requires because there is a delay in the signals getting to your body that it has had enough as when compared to when you eat solid food.

Take control of stress

Stressful activities and environmental conditions can bring about a distortion of the hormonal balance in your body. Major culprits are epinephrine and cortisol. Adrenaline floods the body with a large amount of energy to tackle sudden dangers, while cortisol assists the body in managing stress. These hormones are not meant to be in the body system continuously, they are supposed to be occasionally released. Taking a look at the situation we face every day at the office, home, finances, it is no wonder that the stress levels we face are off the charts. This leads to health problems ranging from obesity to anxiety, cardiac problems to high blood pressure.

To manage the levels of these hormones in the body, stress can be reduced by partaking in yoga, massage, meditation, and treating yourself to some sweet calm music. Make time out during the day to cut down your stress levels no matter how pressed for time you are. It will go a long way in cutting down stress hormones from your body.

Have Quality Sleep Times

The importance of quality of sleep cannot be overestimated. You can exercise regularly and eat a balanced diet, but once your sleep time suffers, all the advantages you could have derived from your diet and exercises will be negated. Sleep deprivation causes an imbalance in the hormones leptin, ghrelin, insulin, and the hormone responsible for growth, most especially in children.

The human body needs to have quality sleep, and the duration should not be taken for granted too. A normal sleep cycle has five stages that must be completed for the release of beneficial hormones. An uninterrupted sleep time of seven hours is needed every day.

Eat Eggs

For nutrition, eat eggs, which are a source of most of the nutrients needed by the body. Eggs increase the levels of PYY and reduce the amount of grehlin and insulin. Eggs can be eaten at any time, but they typically form a part of our breakfast menu. No part of the egg should be left out in favor of the other as both the egg white and the yolk function in sync with each other to reap all the benefits of the hormones that they affect.

Eat Reasonably

Finding a perfect balance between not overeating and eating too much is needed in dealing with weight problems and tackling hormonal issues. When you overeat, there is bound to be a reduction in insulin sensitivity and an increase in insulin levels, especially if you are dealing with weight problems. If you undereat, your body will undergo stress as it tries to deal with the changes. This will lead to an increase in the cortisol levels, which aids weight gain. The goal here is to consume the appropriate calorie intake for your body type to assist you in achieving your optimum weight.

Fiber Diet

Soluble fiber should is an essential part of whatever form of nutrition you eat each day. With a constant intake of this healthy form of fibers, there will be a commensurate increase in the production of hormones and insulin sensitivity. Insoluble fibers also play a major role in regulating the appetite, increase GLP-1, and PYY levels.

CHAPTER THREE

Ways of Carrying out Carb Cycling

Why is Carb Cycling Important?

For starters, it is essential to have some knowledge of how your health will be affected by long and short term calorie and carbohydrate restriction diets. In the short term, your body can function quite well when a diet short on some nutrients is practiced. In the long run, however, your body will go through massive changes and stress that will leave in its wake health challenges that you never bargained for. Taking a look at it critically, when you forget to eat once in a while due to your schedule, your body will not suffer from it, and it can actually be of advantage to your health. There are some forms of fasting that are short and not regular that offer the body massive benefits. If the restriction of nutrients becomes more prolonged and frequent, the effects on the system may not be so desirable.

Due to the connected nature of the body's hormonal system and other organs, any nutritional effect will be felt by every part of the body. If there is a long term nutrient restriction, the likely outcomes are and not limited to fluctuating leptin levels, reduced metabolic rates, heightened physical activity, thyroid hormone release, etc.

If you aim to consume high levels of carb at stipulated times, your body system will never get into a critical state of deprived nutrition. This doesn't mean that you can't get to lose fat, you can as long as the calorie intake is less than what you burn; if there is a calorie deficit. On high carb days, there is an elevated release of the thyroid, which suppresses the hunger pangs. Controlling how you take in carbs also goes a long way in improving the effects of insulin, which is an anabolic hormone. This hormone is responsible for the passage of glucose and amino acid into the cells of the muscle. Without an increase in the levels of insulin in the body, you won't derive the advantage of its anabolic effects. As long as you have a well-regulated plan to increase the levels of insulin with corresponding high carb consumption, you will be able to reap all the advantages of insulin to your body.

How to Carb Cycle

To begin with carb cycling, you have to pick an approach that suits you. Every individual has their peculiarities, and there is no wrong or right when it comes to selecting a plan. Whichever carb cycling technique you pick will be determined by your end goal. For muscle gain, a strategic carb cycling involving 3 low carb days and 4 high carb days might work well for you. For weight loss, on the other hand, 2 days of high carb and 5 days of low carb will be sufficient.

A "normal" carb cycling approach will see you modifying your calorie intake for six days of the week. On the last day of the week, you get to eat whatever you want without keeping a close eye on what you eat.

Ascertain your calorie and carb needs

With this diet plan, men are to consume a maximum of 1,500 calories each day, and ladies have an allocation of 1,200 calories per day when on the low carb days. The number of calories consumed on high carb days will be a bit higher compared to the low carb days. The carb intake on high carb days should be approximately 1.5 grams for every pound of your weight.

Even Day Spread

There is the need to maintain equilibrium in all aspects of the diet, which includes having an even balance in alternating the high and low carb days. You should avoid having a high carb day immediately following a high carb day or a low carb day following a low carb day. Ensure that you alternate the days evenly. If your aim is to lose some weight, which will mean you have to undergo two days of high carb and five days of low carb, do not lump the two days of high carb together. You can put a two days interval between the two high carb days to ensure that your body is not tired out quickly, and you have a regular supply of carbs during this period.

Formulating a meal plan

You can't begin this diet without having an appropriate meal plan, or what will be the essence of going on a carb cycling diet without a well structured eating pattern during the phase? There should be a well laid out plan for your meals for each day of the week. Having a meal plan will guide you and ensure that you keep to the guidelines of the diet as you aim to achieve your goals.

Keeping Records

This will help you monitor how far you are progressing with the diet and checking if your goals are being met or if there needs to be any slight adjustments. After carrying out the diet plan for some time and you notice that you are not making the desired progress, going through your record will assist you in tweaking some variables to come out with a pattern that might just work better than the previous one. Let's say you have been on a low carb diet for four days and a high carb diet for three days and your aim is to lose weight, you can make a change to five days of low carbs and two days of high carb.

The types and forms of nutrition you eat on your low and high carb days are fundamental. The carbs, protein, and fats should all be healthy forms because if they are not good enough, the whole purpose of the dieting would have been defeated.

Consulting your Medical Practitioner

With any diet plan, you should always have a talk with your doctor before starting it. Going on a low carb diet can actually be of advantage to persons who are suffering from pre-existing medical conditions. However, if you are managing an ailment or are in some physiological states that any change in your diet might lead to unwanted results, getting professional advice is the right way to go. As with a change in diet, it also applies to any change that you might want to carry out to how you live your life. Changes to the way we live, eat, and relate to the environment will have upsides and downsides.

The Good Carb

This diet type gives you free rein over what you can eat, it is not restrictive about your intakes. This doesn't mean that when you eat carbs that you shouldn't consume healthy carbs. You should always try as much as you can to consume whole carbs that have not undergone any form of processing or a little processing. The best types of carbohydrates are the complex carbs with a low glycemic index and are high in fiber. These foods, when eaten, will keep the hunger pangs away because it takes a longer time for it to be digested. Some of such carbohydrates include whole-grain foods, potatoes, legumes, etc.

Cheat once in a while

If you don't take the occasional break to indulge in your wild gastrointestinal fantasies, you will most likely fall off the wagon. The diet would seem to be a chore, boring, and ultimately you won't get to enjoy the process as much as you should. This indulgence should be reasonably regular; at least one day a week will do just nicely to keep you going on with the diet. This is not gate free pass to stuff yourself; you should aim to eat reasonably. While eating, be in the moment, eat mindfully, taste, and let every morsel glide over your taste buds. Enjoy it.

Eat in the Morning

You may assume that since you are on a carb cycling diet and on a low carb day, you can take a rain check on breakfast to reduce the number of calories you consume for that day. You should not do that. Don't miss your breakfast, no matter the day of the week. Due to your busy schedule, it might be a chore trying to put something together in the morning; you can have a relatively simple breakfast that won't take much time to put together. Having your breakfast is an integral part of the weight loss process and staying healthy.

Identify the Challenges

The carb cycling diet has as some of its goals to negate the detrimental effects that can come up from the consumption of low carbs for a period of time. With cutting back on any major macros, some adverse side effects are to be expected, which should prompt an immediate restrategizing of the carb cycling routine to bring about an equilibrium of the nutrients that you consume. Some of the expected physical effects include and not limited to extreme fatigue, foul breath, excessive stooling, headaches, etc.

Getting a Grip on What Carb Cycling is

Carb cycling despite its slightly rigid schedule is meant to go easy on the body. As with all classes of nutrients, carbohydrates are also essential to the normal functioning of the human body. Cutting out carbs for a long time from your diet will have disastrous consequences. This is where carb cycling comes in because it provides an adequate supply of the much-needed carbs to the body during this phase. Carbs provide energy for the body, and a restriction of this can result in a slowing metabolic rate causing the body to go into hibernation mode in order to save the available energy.

Calorie Cycling is Carb Cycling

During high carb days, when you consume a higher amount of carbs, you are at the same time taking in a large number of calories. There is no problem with this so long as the carbs are all healthy and wholesome. Carbohydrates have a large amount of calories packed into them. With low carb days, you consume more of foods that don't have as much calories as carbohydrates.

You might have had the mindset that your weight loss will be a problem because of the number of carbs you consume on the high carb days. You should worry less because with the intake of healthy carbs on those days, the little excess carbs will not cause any weight gains.

Foods to Eat and Avoid

Cycling your carbs between high and low carbohydrates intake confers a lot of benefits to your health in addition to substantial weight loss. It is a no brainer that certain classes of foods containing high carbs are to be done away with e.g., highly processed foods, bread, carbonated soft drinks, etc.

With so many mouthwatering and tasteful foods all around, it can be a headache deciding on which should be cut back on. Some of these foods are quite good for the body, but for this diet plan, they won't fit in at all because of the concentration of carbs packed into the food.

The determining factor on the type of foods that you will eat is the number of carbs that you have set to consume for any particular day. During the low carb phase of your carb cycling, limit or control the consumption of the following foods;

Vegetables that contain a lot of starch e.g., sweet potatoes, beets, corn, etc

Bread; whole wheat bread, bagel, white bread, flour tortilla, rice

Certain types of cereals

Sweetened yogurt

Low-fat dressings and fat- free salad dressings

Sugar or honey e.g., Maple syrup, white sugar, agave nectar

Certain types of fruits; raisins, banana, dates, pear, mango, etc.

Beer

Pasta

Fruit or vegetable juice

Legumes; black beans, lentils, peas, kidney beans, pinto beans, etc.

Gluten free baked products

Crackers and Chips

Foods to eat when Carb Cycling

Just as there are certain foods that you limit when you are on the low carb phase, there are foods that are best for the program as a whole. The carbs to consume should be complex, able to control the blood sugar levels and provide the energy needed for daily activities. Food classes already treated above are perfect sources of high carbs that undergo digestion slowly, not undergone any form of processing, and have high fiber contents. These are the good carbs which you should have reasonable amounts during your meals. On the other hand, bad carbs which consist mainly of white flour, highly processed and contains very little amount of fiber.

CHAPTER FOUR

Meal Planning

The setting up of a meal schedule and the types of meals to be had during the carb cycling should have as its backbone sustainability and discipline. You have to stick with the meal plan in order to reap the benefits.

I am a fan of the two days of low carb and one day of high carb intake. During the first two days, you consume foods with low carb contents, or you can also eat foods with high carb contents but in very little amount. On the one day of high carb intake, you can then refuel on really high good carb foods such as brown rice, quinoa, potatoes, yam, etc. After this first three days, you then move onto another two days of low carbs followed by another one-day of high carb with a rest on the seventh day. This meal plan should continue for a minimum of one month, and for optimum results, you should embrace the following guides.

Eat regularly, at least five times a day

You have been inundated with facts about eating too much been one of the major causes of been overweight. This is a wrong idea that has been put to rest by a lot of research with positive results. Having several meals a day that are eaten within stipulated time frames will improve your hormonal balance to a restriction in calorie intake when you consume several reasonably sized portions of meals within a twenty-four hours time frame. This prevents you from getting hungry, which is activated by the hormone cortisol. When the hunger phase becomes a constant in your daily life, with the presence of cortisol always in your body, the body will be forced to increase its level of fat reserves. Having regular small portions of meals throughout the day will cut out the unwanted effects of cortisol and other detrimental levels of hormones that are not needed for your weight loss program.

Whole foods

Eating unprocessed foods is a must for healthy leaving on any diet type. It might be hard getting pocket-friendly whole foods. If you search enough, however, you will get a constant supply of wholesome, nutritious foods.

Fiber

Try as much as you can to eat foods containing a healthy amount of fiber during your meals. Fibers are essential in regulating body weight and blood sugar.

Protein

It is imperative that you eat at least 30 grams of protein at every meal. Protein is an important macronutrient that helps with the building and maintenance of muscle mass, regulation of blood sugar, and also plays an active part in stopping your body from sliding into a catabolic phase, which is most likely to occur once there is an available of carbs into the system.

Omega 3 Fatty Acids

The constant intake of omega 3 fatty acids in your meals will help with the building and maintenance of the composition of the body. This fat and other healthy fats play a crucial role in maintaining the equilibrium of hormones in the body at all times and, most especially, during this dieting program.

The Stumbling Blocks

With any program that you are stepping into, there is the probability that a lot of the factors involved might be unknown to you. Having an in-depth knowledge of the variables that will determine the outcome of your journey is a vital part of the process. For the carb cycling program, here are some of the obstacles that you need to look out for and avoid.

Plan your meals

If you don't make adequate preparations on what you will eat at specified times, your schedule will be thrown into chaos. You might have a lot on your table, work, family issues, and other appointments, your meals should also take priority. You should not let the day's activities compel you into eating junk food that won't do your health any good.

Eat your calories

When you drink your calories through carbonated drinks and other highly concentrated drinks, you will overshoot your daily requirements of calorie intake. In order to achieve and maintain your calorific goals, take more of natural fluids that have not undergone processing e.g., green or black tea, water, and coffee.

Make use of spices

Spices are medicinal and have a lot of health benefits. They play major roles in regulating blood pressure and sugar, weight, and other advantages. So to add flavors to your meals, stay away from artificial flavoring agents, salad dressings, ketchup, sauces, etc.

CHAPTER FIVE

Setting up the Carb Cycling Sample Diet Plan

Though there will be slight individual variations when it comes to setting up a diet plan, the main features will still remain.

The No Carb Days

The carbohydrate intake will be lower than thirty grams per day.

The healthy fat consumption should be at a maximum of about 1 gram/pound of your body weight.

The protein contents of your meals should approximately be at about two grams/pound of body weight.

The Low Carb Days

The carb content should be at 0.5 grams for every pound of your body weight.

The protein content should be 1.5 grams per pound of body weight.

The healthy fat content should be fixed for 0.30 grams for every pound of body weight.

The Moderate Carb Days

Carb content should be 1.5 grams for every pound of your body weight.

The protein content should be at most 1.2 grams for every pound of body weight.

The healthy fat intake should be at 0.2 grams for every pound of body weight.

The High Carb Days

Carb consumption is fixed at a maximum of 2.5 grams for every pound of body weight.

Protein intake is at about a gram for every pound of body weight.

The fat will be at a maximum of 0.15 gram per pound of your body weight.

This is the first step in setting up your daily nutrient intake in the carb cycling diet. After you have this out of the way, what you should now tackle is the type of foods that enjoy that will fit into the bill of healthy foods.

Sample High Carb Diet Plan

Breakfast - two large organic eggs scrambled in extra virgin olive oil, a cup of oats with a banana, and a cup of green tea.

Lunch – chicken burgers made from your kitchen, one apple, 2 rice cakes

Snack – one medium-sized baked sweet potato with two grilled salmon fillet and some green vegetables.

Exercise Meal – 3 tablespoons of protein powder, 1 cup of mixed berries, 2 medium-sized bananas, and 1 cup of almond milk.

Dinner – half grilled boneless duck breast with one cup cooked quinoa and grilled lentils.

This diet plan is perfect for a day in which you are planning to exercise and go through some rigorous physical activities.

Sample Low Carb Diet Plan

Breakfast – five whole organic eggs scrambled in coconut oil with half a cup of kale, one cup protein shake.

Lunch – hamburgers with kale, eggplant and parsley salad, a handful of roasted peanuts.

Snack – 2 small boiled Irish potatoes with half a cup of mixed vegetables and Parmesan cheese.

Dinner – half a pound of grilled ham with some olives, grilled Brussels sprouts and lentils, and a tablespoon of coconut oil.

This meal plan fits in nicely for a day with no physical exertion expected.

The carb diet plan gives preference to a relatively high intake of protein while you alter the levels of carbs that you consume depending on your level of activity on any given day. It provides a balance to your daily diet by making sure that you eat the right amounts of both the essential micronutrients and macronutrients. With a well balanced and followed diet plan, there will be positive changes in your health in a few weeks.

This diet plan is simple and easy to set up, but at the same time, you have to employ a high level of discipline. When you are on a high carb day, your level of fat consumption will be low, and when you are on a low carb day, your level of fat intake will be high. This alteration will put your body into a calorie deficit, which will ultimately result in weight loss.

With carb cycling, there is no need to keep an absolute record or track of your calorie intake, all you need to do is keep to the guidelines of the diet plan, and you will do just fine. This makes it easier for a lot of individuals to embrace and practice this diet plan.

Carb Cycling Diet for Body Composition Maintenance or Muscle Building

With the loss of fat, a lot of us want to bulk up with rippling muscles at the same time. If this is your goal, you will need to make adjustments to your macronutrient and calorie intake. For this process in a seven day week, the high carb days should be for four days while the low carb days should fill in the remaining three days. The days of low carb will cut back on the ability of the body to retain water, which is why you will appear lean. The low carb days will also improve your appetite to consume more protein and fatty foods.

To solve the problem of what to eat on which day, I have compiled a list of foods to help you.

High Carb Fruits

Melons

Banana

Pineapple

Oranges

Blueberries

Apples

Cherries

Mango

Pear

Kiwi

Grapefruit

Raisin

High Carb Grains

Quinoa

Brown rice

Pasta

White rice

Oats

Barley

Whole grain bread

High Carb Vegetables

Corn

Beets

pumpkin

Brussels sprouts

Sweet potatoes

Peas

Lima beans

White potatoes

I will layout a diet plan for one week, which will provide you with all the nutrients and variety needed to make this journey a worthwhile experience.

Day 1

Low carb

Breakfast – grapefruit, pear, and mango salad with some mixed berries and yogurt.

Snack – one large banana

Lunch – brown rice salad, combined with sliced eggplant, 3 hardboiled whole organic eggs, 1 large tomato.

Snack – 1 large apple, one handful of almond nuts

Dinner – Stir fry boneless chicken breasts in extra virgin olive oil, 1 teaspoon chopped ginger, 1 cup mixed greens, ½ cup finely chopped carrots, 1 small onion; chopped, add 1 teaspoon of soy sauce and ¼ cup water. Stir well and allow to cook for a few minutes over low to medium heat. Serve with 1 cup of cooked brown rice.

Snack – 2 rice cakes

Daily totals: 1870 calories, 221 carbs, 110g protein, 70g fat

Day 2

Low carb

Breakfast – seed mixture, combine 3 tablespoons of sunflower seeds, sesame seeds, pumpkin seeds and oats in a bowl, add some water, and soaked in milk for at least an hour or all through the night by placing it in a fridge. Serve with 3 tablespoons of full cream yogurt and one large grated apple.

Snack – 1 large banana and some roasted peanuts

Lunch – 1 pita bread made from wholemeal flour with sardine, cheddar cheese, and 1 teaspoon of coconut oil.

Snack – a slice of watermelon

Dinner – zesty cod steak; apply some extra virgin olive oil to the cod steak; sprinkle some salt, pepper, and other spices of your choice on it. Squeeze half a lemon over the fish and grill in for ten to fifteen minutes. Serve warm with 3 cups of steamed mixed vegetables.

Snack – 1 grapefruit

Daily totals: 1798 calories, 168 carbs, 138g protein, 84g fat

Day 3

High Carb

Breakfast – add 65g of oats to a cup of water and cook over low to medium heat. Before it is done cooking, add 220g of frozen mixed berries and combine well for another three minutes. Serve warm with some yogurt.

Snack – 1 apple

Lunch – 1 large baked sweet potato with 2 tablespoons hummus, a thinly sliced small onion, a small sliced green bell pepper, 1 small sliced cherry tomatoes, and some vegetables of your choice.

Snack – 1 slice wholewheat bread and one large apple

Dinner – apply some extra virgin olive oil to a large salmon fillet. Spice it up with some salt, ginger and garlic powder, black pepper. Grill it for ten to fifteen minutes. Serve with 220g of boiled white potatoes, 150g steamed carrots, Brussels sprouts, and some kale.

Snack – quinoa cakes

Daily totals: 1811 calories, 335g carbs, 74g protein, 38g fat

Day 4

Low carb

Breakfast – whisk four large organic whole eggs with a small chopped onion, one small thinly sliced bell pepper, 3 tablespoon yogurt, black pepper, and salt. Cook on low to medium heat. Add to a low to carb-free tortilla. One cup of black coffee.

Snack – one large apple and half a cup of sunflower seeds

Lunch – a cup of brown beans with one large salmon fillet. 3 cups of mixed vegetables with a dash of extra virgin olive oil, apple cider vinegar, and salt.

Snack – tangerine

Dinner – one large roasted turkey breast with a cup of chopped carrot, one small thinly sliced onion, one crushed garlic clove, one teaspoon minced ginger, a teaspoon of black pepper. Serve warm and enjoy.

Snack – 70g of grapes and one small banana.

Daily totals: 1790 calories, 152 carbs, 153g protein, 73g fat

Day 5

Low Carb

Breakfast – 3 large wholesome organic hardboiled eggs, 1 slice toasted pita bread with a tablespoon of butter

Snack – one pear and one handful of grapes

Lunch – halibut and avocado pear: combine one avocado and 2 large grilled halibut fillet with a teaspoon of vinegar and spices. Serve with a side of

1 small grated carrot, ½ a tomato, 1 small sliced eggplant, 1 cup chopped kale

Snack – 3 oatcakes with some cheese

Dinner – tuna ratatouille: sauté a teaspoon of chopped ginger, one clove minced garlic, one small thinly sliced onion in one tablespoon of extra virgin olive oil. Introduce one small chopped carrot and pepper, two large chopped tomatoes and one can of tuna. Cook over low to medium heat for 8 – 10 minutes. Serve warm and enjoy.

Snack – one medium-sized banana and a handful of nuts.

Daily totals: 1792 calories, 162 carbs, 129g protein, 79g fat

Day 6

High Carb

Breakfast – combine 6 tablespoons of yogurt, 220g of mixed frozen berries, 1 tablespoon honey, and 1 cup of oats.

Snack – 1 pita bread topped with ½ onion thinly sliced, 1 small tomato sliced and cheddar cheese.

Lunch – Quinoa salad: combine a mixture of salad vegetables that you desire. Add 1 cup of quinoa, two tablespoons of extra virgin olive oil and one teaspoon of apple cider vinegar.

Snack – 5 oatcakes with unsalted butter and one banana

Dinner – spice a boneless chicken breast and grill for 10 to 15 minutes. Serve with steamed cauliflower, 100g of lentils, and 50g of wild rice.

Daily totals: 1895 calories, 256 carbs, 128g protein, 48g fat

CHAPTER SIX

The Ultimate Food List

Discussed and listed out in this chapter are foods that should be avoided, consumed with caution, and eaten regularly. This list of foods should be adhered to and act as a template with your carb cycling food program to derive the maximum benefits.

Vegetables 3- 5 servings every day

Eat regularly

Avocados

Broccoli

Sprouts

Cabbage

Bok choy

Olives

Mustard greens

Sauerkraut

Swiss chard

Nori

Eat with Caution

Potatoes

Peas

Yams

Plantains

Corn

Carrots

Sweet potatoes

Zucchini

Celery

Red lettuce

Squash

Radishes

Romaine lettuce

Stay Away From

Unwashed vegetables

Non-organic vegetables

Canned vegetables

Carbohydrates

Eat Regularly

Sprouted legumes

Quinoa

White or brown rice

Full fat yogurt

Eat with Caution

Raw seeds

Millet

Sprouted or soaked wheat produce

Soaked legumes

Stay Away From

Roasted nuts and seeds

Common wheat produce

Soybeans

Canned legumes

Regular yogurt

Fava beans

Scones

Cookies

Bread

Crackers

Cereal

Bagels

Healthy Fats

Eat Regularly

Extra virgin olive oil

Coconut oil

Olives

Macadamia nut oil

Full fat organic yogurt

Organic grass-fed butter

Sardines, wild salmon, tilapia, trout

Organic eggs

Pure cod liver oil

Eat with Caution

Almond butter

Raw nuts

Bacon

Peanut butter

Palm oil

Dark chocolate

Coconut ice cream

Cold-press flax oil

Stay Away From

Roasted seeds

Cottonseed oil

Soy ice cream

Regular butter

Regular ice cream

Commercial salad dressings

Margarine

Canola oil

Farmed fish

Milk chocolate

Protein 2 -4 servings every day

Eat Regularly

Grass-fed beef

Organic pork

Sardine

Wild salmon

Protein powder

Tilapia

Full fat organic yogurt

Eat with Caution

Organic cottage cheese

Raw cheese

Yogurt cheese

Soaked or sprouted legumes or beans

Raw nut butter

Miso

Dried meats

Raw seeds and nuts

Stay Away From

Chemically preserved meats

Non-organic dairy produce

Protein powders with preservatives

Commercially processed meats

Tofu

Canned legumes and beans

Roasted nut butter

Fruits 1 – 2 servings per day

Eat Regularly

Grapefruit

Apples

Peach

Apricots

Pears

Berries

Cherries

Bananas

Oranges

Mangoes

Papayas

Nectarines

Watermelon

Pineapples

Eat with Caution

Grapes

Lemons

Limes

Figs

Fruit juices

Strawberries

Dried fruits

Dates

Stay Away From

Packed dried fruits

Fruits in syrup

Canned fruits

Sugar-coated dried fruits

Fruit candy

Spices, herbs, and Sweeteners

Eat Regularly

Allspice

Cinnamon

Fennel

Xylitol

Turmeric

Garlic

Ginger

Cumin

Cloves

Stevia

Maltitol

Eat with Caution

Natural fruit sweetener

Maple syrup

Molasses

Raw honey

Red pepper

Truvia

Apple cider vinegar

Fermented soy sauce

Stay Away From

Regular honey

Aspartame

Candy

Agave syrup

Processed sugar

MSG

Other Books by the Author

The Healing Path with Essential CBD oil and Hemp oil: The Simple Beginner's Guide to Managing Anxiety Attacks, Weight Loss, Diabetes and Holistic Healing

Suffering from arthritis, diabetes, severe chronic pain and a host of other debilitating ailments can limit your quality of life. The constant intake of a cocktail of medications will always leave you with horrible aftermaths that were not listed on the package of such drugs. The battering and deterioration that your internal organs undergo can only just be imagined as these medications cause more damage than good in the long run. The wholesome nature and abundant benefits that CBD oil has cannot just be overlooked. Its uses range from managing common pains and to the more complex and debilitating conditions that ravage us in this age and time. It is used for the treatment of pains, depression, irritable bowel syndrome, epilepsy and illnesses that you can never imagine will be easily handled by this compound. CBD is wholly naturally without any hint of synthetic compounds is just what you need for that immediate relief from the condition that has been keeping you down for so long. This book is a beginner guide on what CBD and Hemp oil are, all you need to know, some of the numerous ailments that it can be used to treat, modes of preparation, how to dose on CBD and a guide of how to shop for CBD. Also addressed in this book is the nagging issues of legal barriers that are continually being surmounted with each passing day as new information on the benefits of CBD oil comes to light.

Are you ready to know how you can use CBD oil to

- Boost your immune system
- Have a clearer skin
- Control those pains
- Increase your sexual appetite

- Lighten your moods
- Have a good night's rest
- Improve your learning and retention abilities
- And have a generally healthy and wholesome lifestyle?

In this beginner's guide, you will be made aware of how CBD oil can be the best thing that ever happened to you.

So for how long are you going to cope with that pain, the condition that keeps you down most of the day? Take that all critical, decisive step now, dump the medications that are not doing you any good and embrace the natural path to healing. Get this book now!

https://www.amazon.com/dp/B07GY217ZY

Cannabis Bud Smoothie: Healthy Medicinal Drinks and Marijuana Infusions

Quite a lot of folks with chronic medical conditions are sceptical about the consumption of marijuana by smoking it. If you are in this category, then here is an easy way out. Taking in medicinal cannabis by adding it to your delicious smoothies and juicing it will give you all the health benefits and much more! Ingesting of cannabis fresh and raw is the most advantageous as all the nutrients, and cannabinoid compounds will remain intact without undergoing any change into compounds that you may not necessarily need at this point.

You will learn how to incorporate cannabis buds and cannabis infusions into your daily smoothies to aid you in managing those severe pains, inflammations, ailments and generally giving you a more healthy life.

This book is filled with a delicious smoothie, and juice recipes packed loaded with vitamins, nutrients and cannabinoids. The recipes are organic, gluten and sugar-free with the foundation been cannabis.

In this book, you will learn;

- The great health benefits of cannabis
  How to prepare delicious smoothies and juices
- Ease away those excruciating pains
  And so much more!

BUY this book today and begin your journey towards a more healthier life!

https://www.amazon.com/dp/B07MLX2SP3

Cannabis Cultivation and Horticulture: The Simple Guide to Growing Marijuana Indoors Using Hydroponics

This is an excellent guide for beginners and professionals alike on the indoor cultivation of marijuana for personal use using hydroponics and soil. It brings to you the simple techniques and methods need to have a thriving sanctuary for your cannabis plants and produce plants with potent buds and massive amounts of resins! Cultivating your cannabis indoors gives you the opportunity to monitor its growth and make adjustments to the environmental conditions that will significantly stimulate the growth of the plant. It is also an avenue to prevent the pestilence that comes with outdoor cultivation. Looking to have a basic knowledge that can be leveraged to grow great plants? Then this is the book for you!

Major and minor parts involved in the cultivation of cannabis are thoroughly handled. From the design and type of sanctuary space to the kind of nutrients, lightning to temperature, pest control to flow of air; everything you need to grow potent strains of marijuana is just within your grasp. Each stage of cultivation from obtaining the seeds to drying and curing is fully explained in terms that you can easily understand and put to practice immediately.

So do you want to take the first steps towards nurturing this beautiful plant from seed to a potent wonder of nature? This book will teach you how to

- Grow your stash while employing high safety standards
- Learn how to secure a discrete growing space in a confined area
- Have the ability to determine the potency of your product
- Force flowering
- Applying the best nutrients formulas to your plants
- Crossing and identifying the best strain for you
- Getting all unfertilized female plants (Sensimilla)
- Controlling Pests

- Making the best use of the hydroponics
- And so much more!

Getting started with this book will make you an enlightened cultivator and appreciator of everything cannabis and not just a grower. BUY this book now and have a high time!

https://www.amazon.com/dp/B07MC4ZBQT

The Complete Instant Pot Cookbook: Simple Ketogenic Diet Cookbook Recipes, The Simple Slow Cooker Cookbook and The Healthy Crock Pot Cookbook

This amazing collection of books will take you on a journey of culinary delights that you can put together with ease. Coming home to a well cooked, a stomach-warming meal will now be the norm for you and your household. With quite a number of great recipes to choose from you will be absolutely spoilt with choices.

Lay your hand on this volume of healthy crockpot and instant pot recipes for the price of one. You will never have a shortage of recipes you can try out at any given time ranging from desserts to main dishes and chili to exotic recipes. You will not just be getting mouth-watering recipes, also included are guidelines on what to look out for when you want to buy a crockpot, healthy tips on going on a ketogenic diet plan and so much more!

What are you waiting for? Do not let this opportunity slip by you. GET this book NOW and also as a gift for your loved ones.

https://www.amazon.com/dp/B07K88MQPQ

About the Author

Rina S. Gritton has been all about healthy intake of food and living the life of a real food aficionado. With her it is about food, making us of spices, herbs, and other ingredients around in nature that ensures we all stay at the peak of our health at all times.

She has been putting together great recipes and meals as a hobby and business to loved ones and clients alike. What started as a challenge to help her parents and siblings eat better turned to a full-fledged campaign and career in making use of purely organic foods and materials around us.

A dietician with several years experience in the treatment of dietary issues and business owner catering for the desires of folks to have organic and tasteful meals, she also guest writes for blogs, websites, and volunteers in cooking classes in high schools.

She lives in Santa Monica, California with her husband and children.

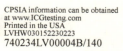

CPSIA information can be obtained
at www.ICGtesting.com
Printed in the USA
LVHW030152230223
740234LV00004B/140